T0131754

MY MUMMY & ME

All About Perinatal Mental Health Problems

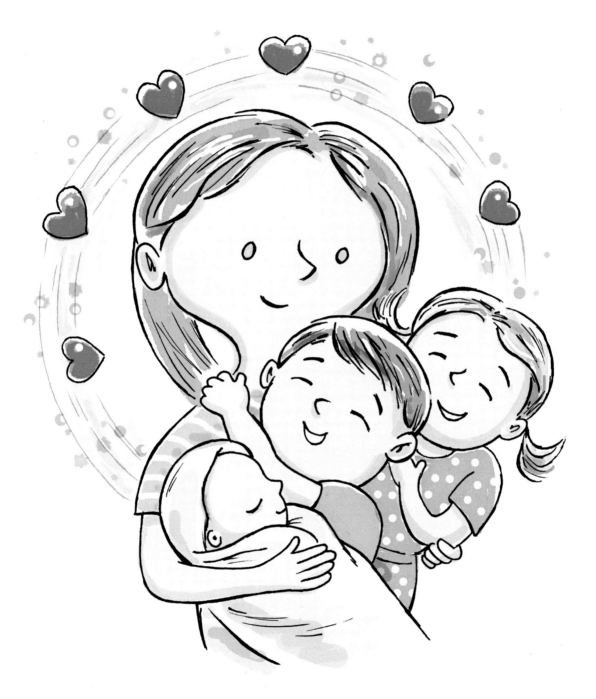

Written by Narelle Mullins & Dr Eleanor Ball

Illustrated by Paul Carter

CAMBRIDGE
UNIVERSITY PRESS

University Printing House, Cambridge CB2 8BS, United Kingdom

One Liberty Plaza, 20th Floor, New York, NY 10006, USA

477 Williamstown Road, Port Melbourne, VIC 3207, Australia

314-321, 3rd Floor, Plot 3, Splendor Forum, Jasola District Centre, New Delhi - 110025, India

79 Anson Road, #06-04/06, Singapore 079906

Cambridge University Press is part of the University of Cambridge.

It furthers the University's mission by disseminating knowledge in the pursuit of
education, learning and research at the highest international levels of excellence.

www.cambridge.org
Information on this title: www.cambridge.org/9781911623007
DOI: 10.1017/9781911623014

© Royal College of Psychiatrists 2018

First published 2018

A catalogue record for this publication is available from the British Library

ISBN 978-1-911-62300-7 Paperback

Cambridge University Press has no responsibility for the persistence or
accuracy of URLs for external or third-party internet websites referred to in
this publication, and does not guarantee that any content on such websites is,
or will remain, accurate or appropriate.

....

Every effort has been made in preparing this book to provide accurate and
up-to-date information which is in accord with accepted standards and practice
at the time of publication. Although case histories are drawn from actual cases,
every effort has been made to disguise the identities of the individuals involved.
Nevertheless, the authors, editors and publishers can make no warranties that the
information contained herein is totally free from error, not least because clinical
standards are constantly changing through research and regulation. The authors,
editors and publishers therefore disclaim all liability for direct or consequential
damages resulting from the use of material contained in this book. Readers
are strongly advised to pay careful attention to information provided by the
manufacturer of any drugs or equipment that they plan to use.

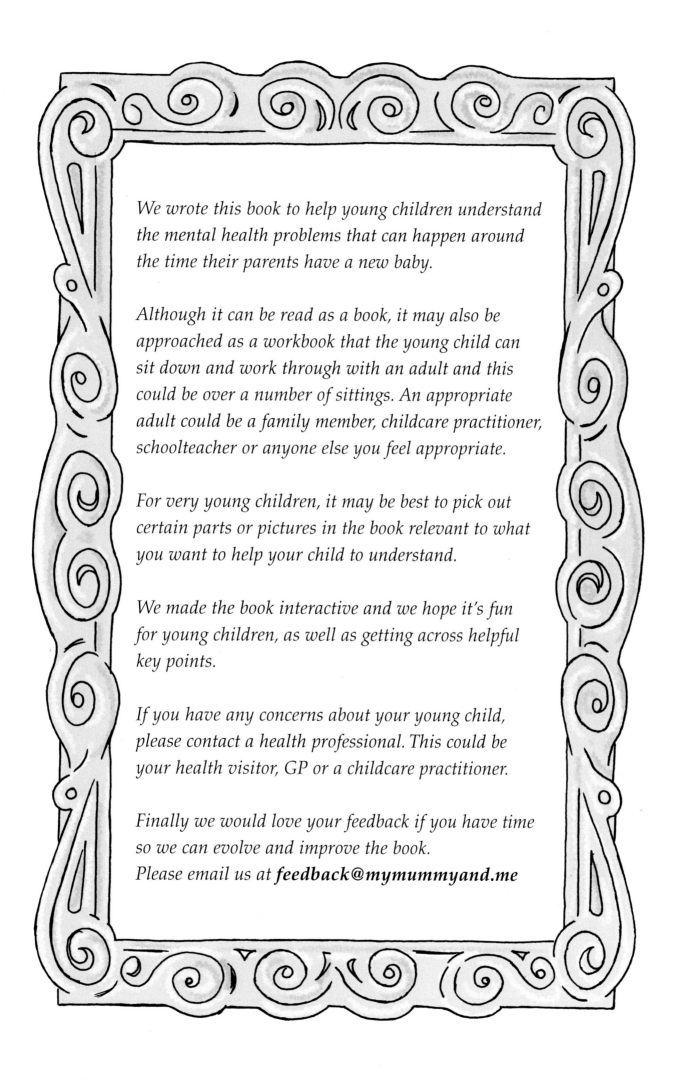

We wrote this book to help young children understand the mental health problems that can happen around the time their parents have a new baby.

Although it can be read as a book, it may also be approached as a workbook that the young child can sit down and work through with an adult and this could be over a number of sittings. An appropriate adult could be a family member, childcare practitioner, schoolteacher or anyone else you feel appropriate.

For very young children, it may be best to pick out certain parts or pictures in the book relevant to what you want to help your child to understand.

We made the book interactive and we hope it's fun for young children, as well as getting across helpful key points.

If you have any concerns about your young child, please contact a health professional. This could be your health visitor, GP or a childcare practitioner.

Finally we would love your feedback if you have time so we can evolve and improve the book.
Please email us at **feedback@mymummyand.me**

Dedicated to Harry, Charlie and all children with mummies who are temporarily not well.

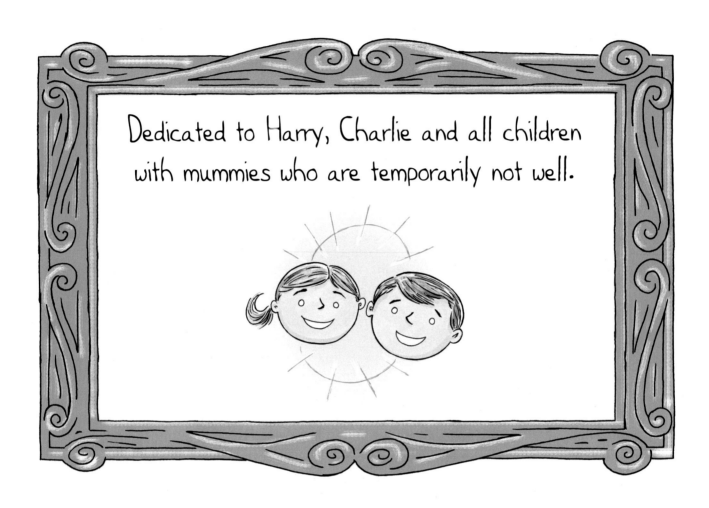

Jamie's Mummy had been different since the new baby arrived.

Jamie noticed she didn't smile as much, wasn't as much fun and sometimes cried.

Jamie also noticed she sometimes did or said strange things.

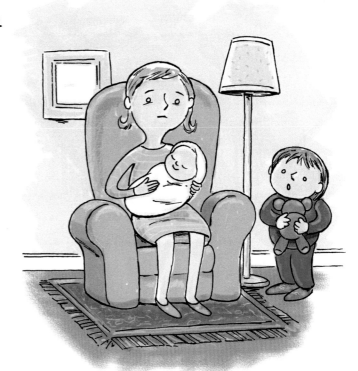

Mummy said it wasn't anybody's fault, she just wasn't feeling well.

She said it was something to do with 'mental health'.

Jamie wanted to know more about mental health so a grown-up sat down to talk with him and here's what Jamie learnt...

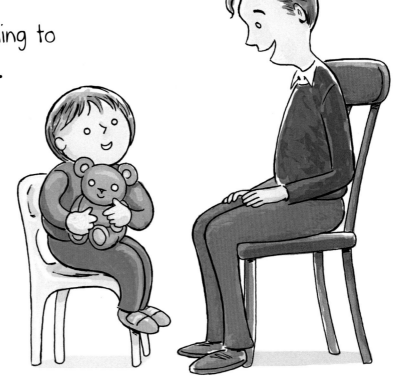

Mental health is to do with how things work inside your brain.

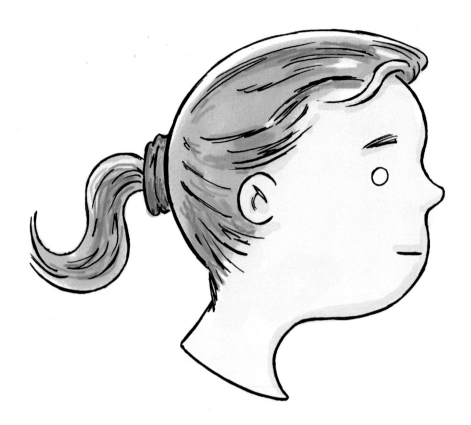

You can't see your brain.
It's inside your head.

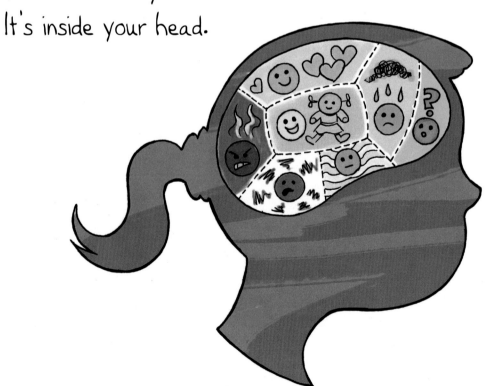

But your brain is very important as it produces feelings.

Here are some examples of feelings:

frustrated **CROSS** **ANGRY** **sad**

You might sometimes feel these if you play a game and you don't win.

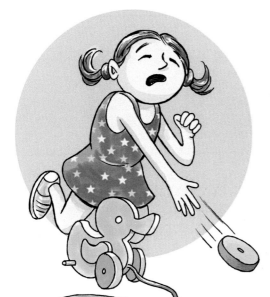

Or perhaps when your toy breaks, you might even cry, shout or throw things.

You might feel some of these feelings when your friends don't want to play with you. You might even hide away and cry.

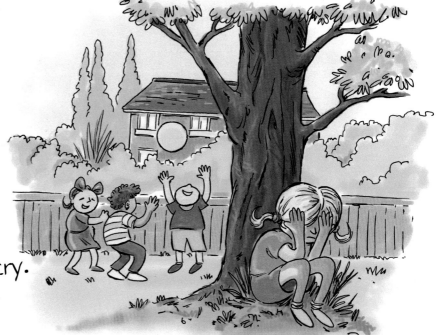

There are lots more feelings you can have, such as feeling excited and happy. Lots of things might make you happy, like playing with your favourite toy.

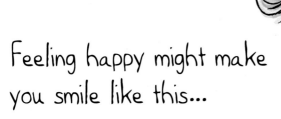

Feeling happy might make you smile like this...

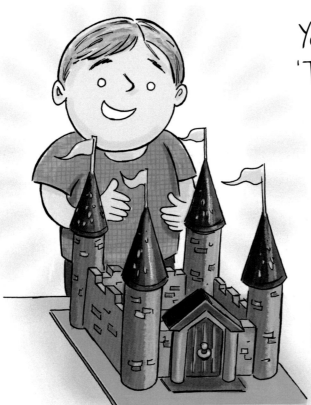

You might think to yourself 'This toy is brilliant'.

That's called a thought.

And all feelings and thoughts happen in your brain.

If you turn the page, you can draw a picture of when you're happy and when Mummy is happy.

When I'm happy:

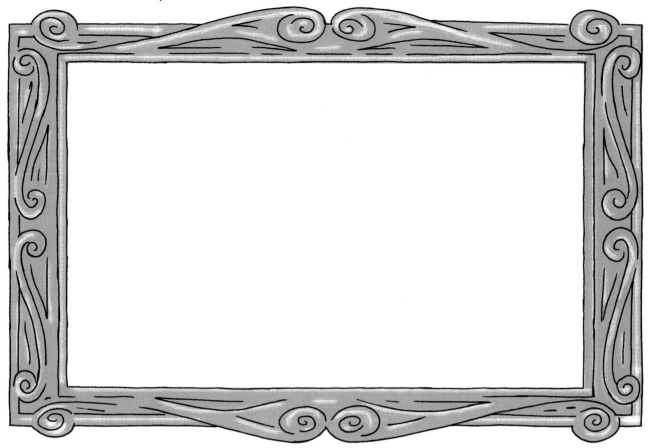

When Mummy is happy:

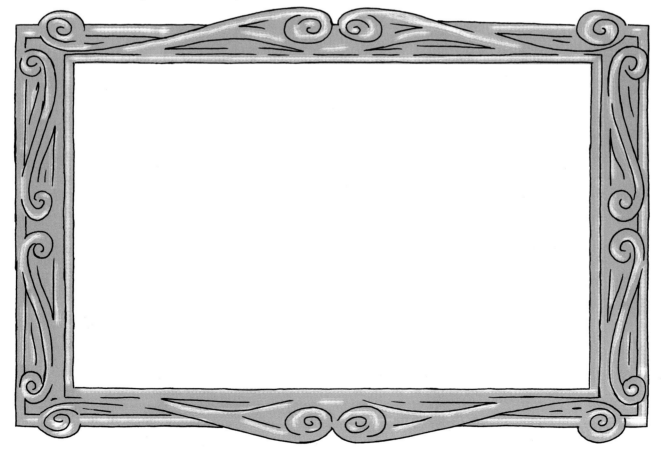

As you can see, there are lots of different feelings a person can have:

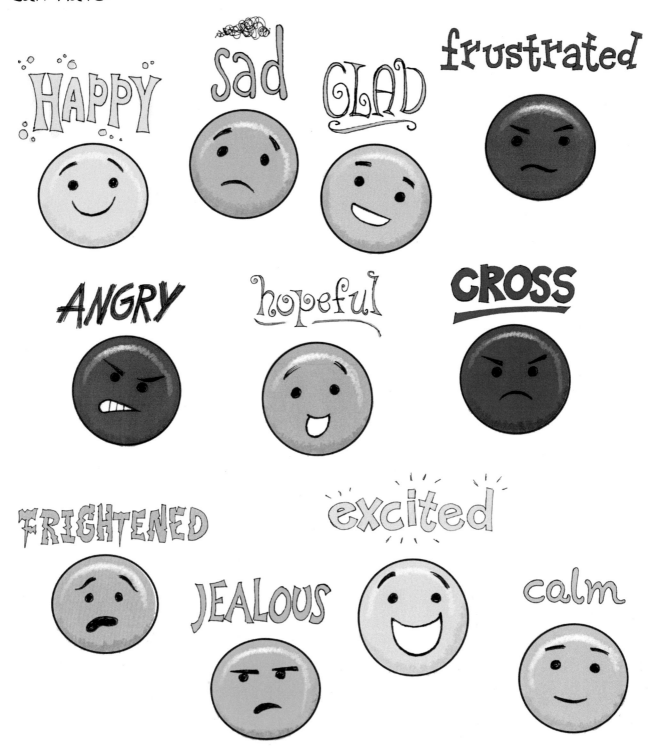

Can you put a tick next to any of the feelings that you've felt before?

You can talk about these feelings if you want to.

When you have the right balance of feelings, your mental health is good.

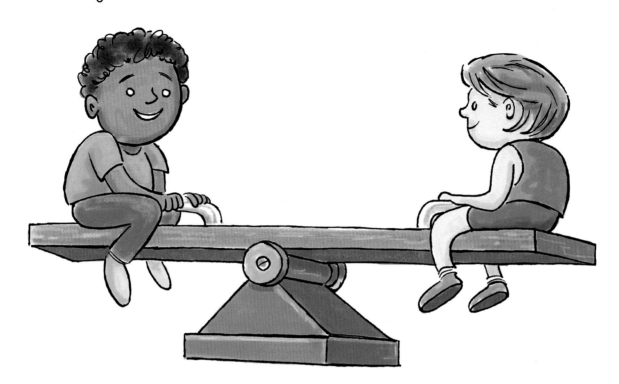

But sometimes our brains can get a bit poorly and thoughts and feelings get all mixed up.

If this happens to Mummy she might feel a certain way for no reason at all.

This can cause problems called 'mental health problems'.

You might hear words like:

Depression **Anxiety** Psychosis Bipolar

And other new words...

These are all mental health problems that are caused when the brain gets a bit poorly. The good news is, with special help, it gets better again.

If Mummy has one of these problems she might seem a bit different.

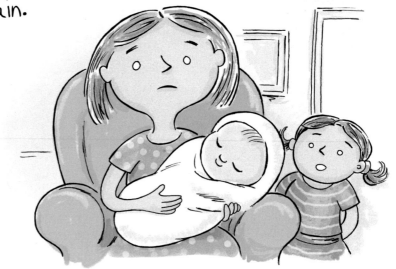

She might look sad or not smile as much. She might even be snappy or find it hard to play and have fun.

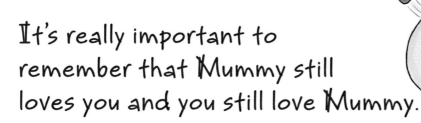

It's really important to remember that Mummy still loves you and you still love Mummy.

There are special people to make Mummy's mental health problem better. They are part of a team that you may hear being called the Perinatal Team.

Here are some of the special people in the team:

... **PSYCHIATRIST**
... **DOCTOR**

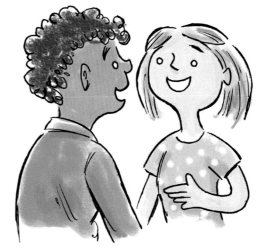

... **PSYCHOLOGIST** ... **NURSE**

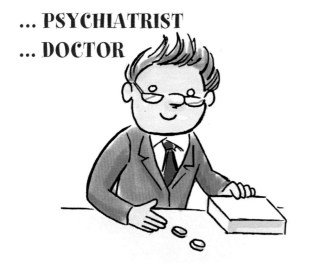

... **SOCIAL WORKER**

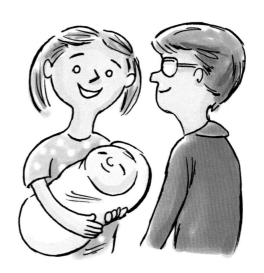

... **NURSERY NURSE** ... **STUDENT**
... **SUPPORT WORKER**

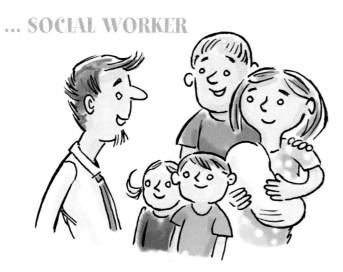

These people may help Mummy by giving her some special medicine or by talking to her. They might also help Mummy look after the new baby.

A social worker helps the family and makes sure everyone is ok.

If Mummy is taking medicines to help her get better, it's important to remember that:

Sometimes the medicines can make Mummy sleepy so Mummy may not be able to talk or play with you as much.

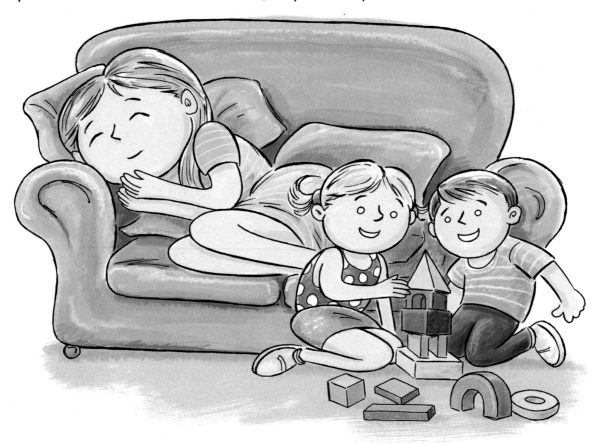

But Mummy still loves you and you still love Mummy.

It can take time for
the medicines to work.

Sometimes it takes
days or weeks.

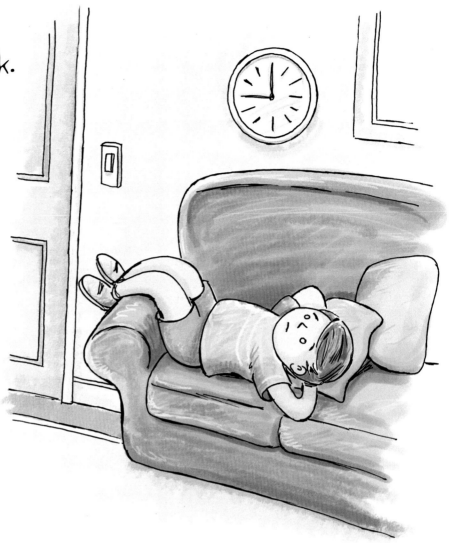

Another important thing about medicines is that children
aren't allowed to touch them.

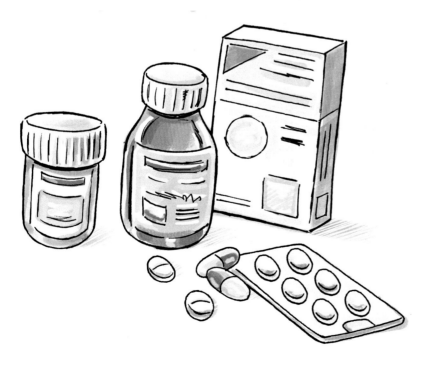

They are dangerous
for children.

But they are safe
for Mummy.

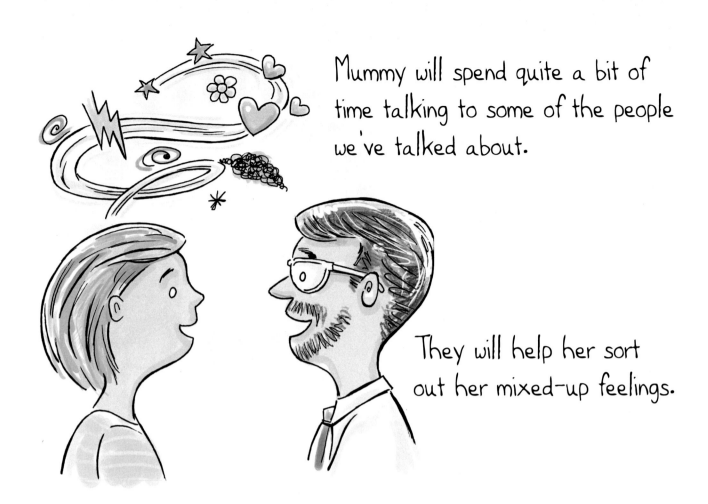

Mummy will spend quite a bit of time talking to some of the people we've talked about.

They will help her sort out her mixed-up feelings.

It takes time to sort out the mixed-up feelings.

Sometimes Mummy may be upset when she's talking to the people helping her but that's ok.

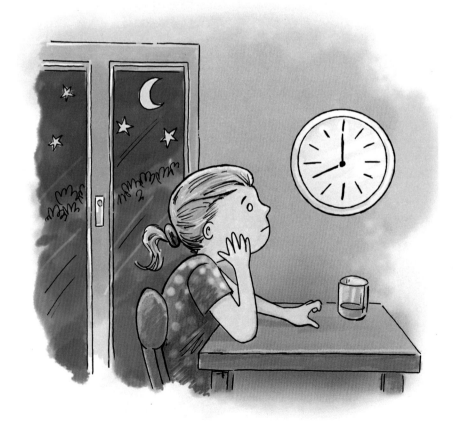

Talking can help the mixed-up feelings get sorted out.

As well as Mummy talking to people, it's good for you to talk to people too.

If you don't understand things or you're worried about anything, it's ok to ask people to explain things to you.

Can you think of anything you want to know right now?

If you think of something later, you could draw it or write it down here and show it to a grown-up.

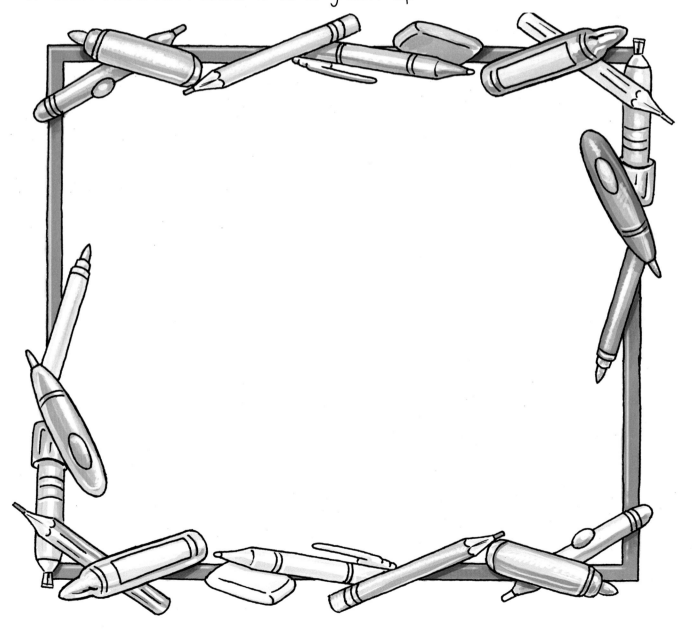

Sometimes Mummy can't stay at home to get better and needs to go to a special place called a Mother and Baby Unit. Here, the Perinatal Team help her get better more quickly.

It's a bit like a hospital but a lot nicer and the baby can stay there too.

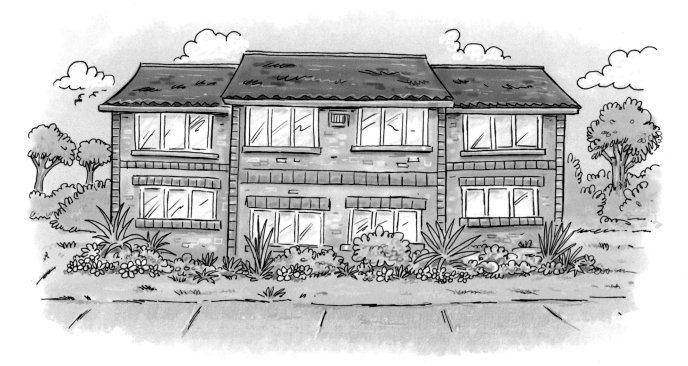

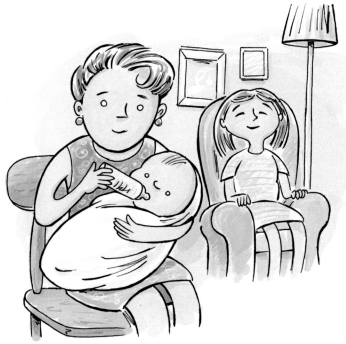

It's good for Mummy to keep the baby with her as there are lots of people that can help with the baby so Mummy can rest.

If your Mummy isn't staying in the Mother and Baby Unit, you can turn to page 19 now.

The Mother and Baby Unit is in a place called

....

Mummy has her own room there and she may have her own bathroom.

She shares a kitchen, dining room and lounge with the other mummies who are there to get better.

There is a nursery for the babies where they can sleep and play.

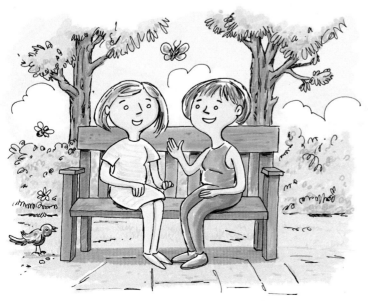

And Mummy will be able to go outside for fresh air.

Here are some words that describe the Mother and Baby Unit:

safe **SECURE** friendly

busy warm comfortable

nurturing supportive

colourful clean

When Mummy is staying at the Mother and Baby Unit, you can ask a grown-up to take you to visit her. They may be the same person that you're staying with.

You can draw them below.

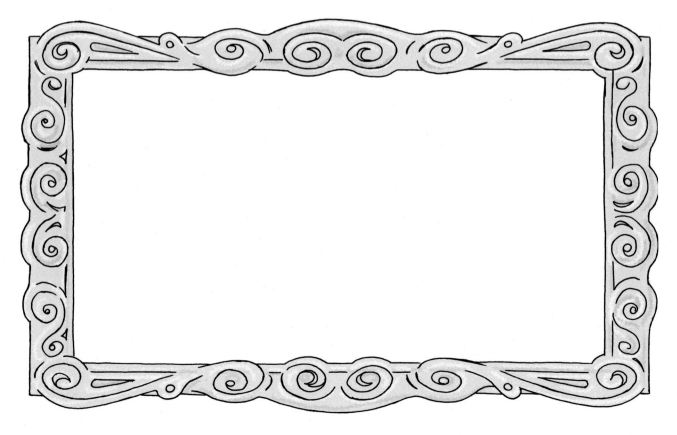

In the Mother and Baby Unit, there are lots of special people who will spend time with Mummy.

They will also help her look after the baby so that she can rest.

You might hear the words Occupational Therapist, too.

This special person may teach Mummy to do different activities to help her feel better.

These activities might include the new baby or they might include you.

Sometimes it can take a while for things to feel like before.

But remember, everyone will be working hard to help Mummy feel better again.

When the time is right, Mummy will come home from the Mother and Baby Unit but she will carry on seeing some of the special people so they can keep making her better.

It's a bit like if you fall over and scrape your knee. You might need a plaster.

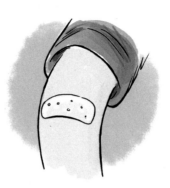

When it's better, you take the plaster off but the mark on your knee might not go for a while.

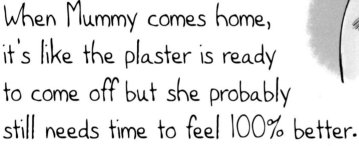

When Mummy comes home, it's like the plaster is ready to come off but she probably still needs time to feel 100% better.

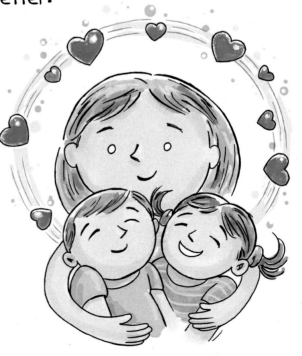

Mummy may still not play or talk with you as much as she used to but remember:

Mummy still loves you and you still love Mummy.

You might want to know a bit more about the people from the Perinatal Team who visit Mummy at home.

If you want to you could fill this in to help you.

The Nurse who visits Mummy is called

....

🚗 Their car is

....

The Doctor who visits Mummy is called

....

🚗 Their car is

....

The Nursery Nurse who visits Mummy is called

....

🚗 Their car is

....

The Social Worker who visits is called

....

and their car is ....

This is our car!

If there are other visitors you can write them down here.

The .... who visits Mummy

is called ....

Their car is ....

The .... who visits Mummy

is called ....

Their car is ....

20

You might feel you want to help Mummy get better but you don't need to worry. Lots of people are helping to do that right now so you can still play and have fun.

You might want to draw or think about some of the things that make you feel happy.

What are the things you like doing with Mummy when she's feeling well?

What things does Mummy do that make you feel happy?

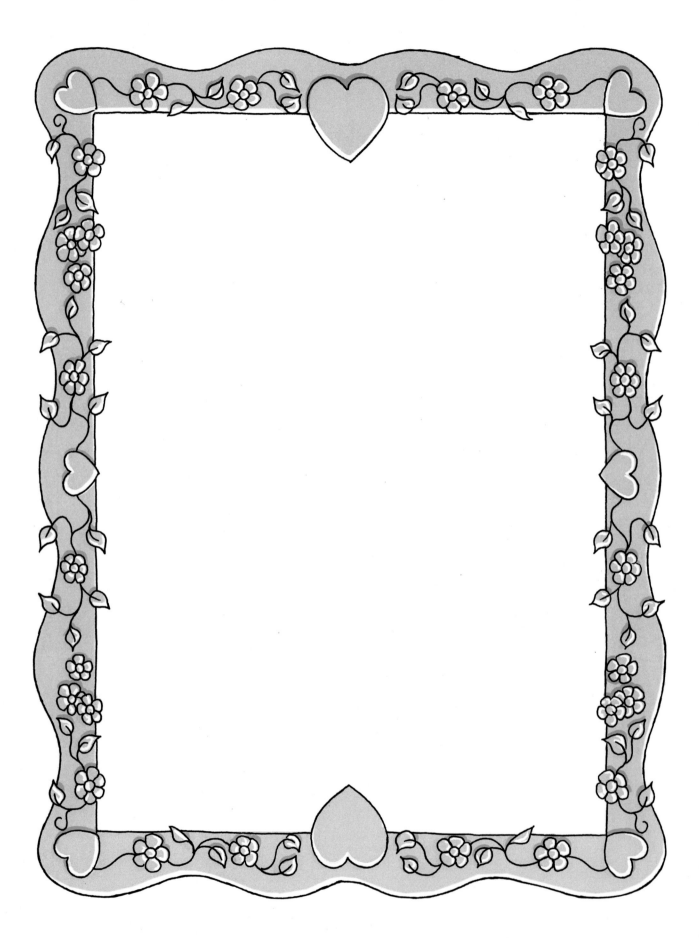

What things do you do that make Mummy feel happy?

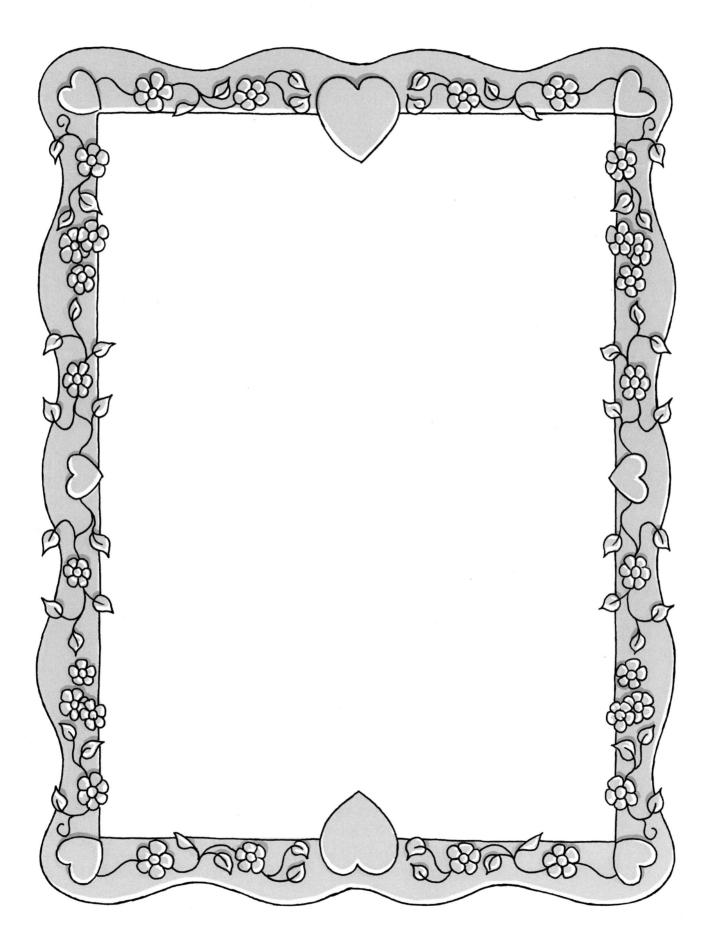

There are other things that might help to make Mummy feel better too. These are:

Resting when she's tired

Letting other grown-ups help her

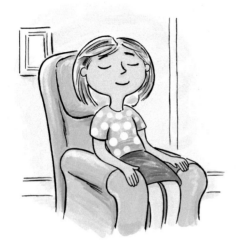
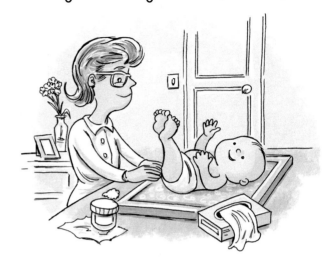

Doing nice things

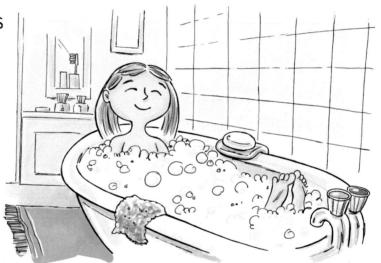

Talking to people

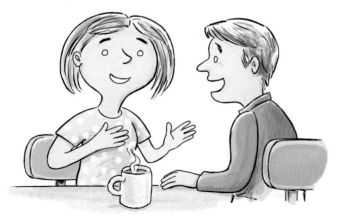
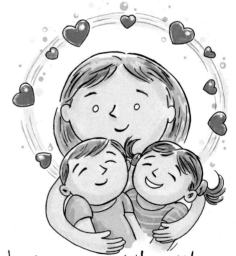

Having a cuddle with you

These are the things that Jamie learnt about mental health. And by reading this book, you've learnt them too.

If your Mummy feels poorly like Jamie's Mummy, here are the important things to remember:

- Mental health problems happen when the brain is a bit poorly
- It's nobody's fault and the problems get better with the help of special people
- You can't catch mental health problems like you can a cold
- Getting better can take time (there are activities at the end of this book if you're bored)
- If Mummy is in the Mother and Baby Unit, it's a nice place for her to be
- If you feel scared or worried then talking to a grown-up is an excellent thing to do

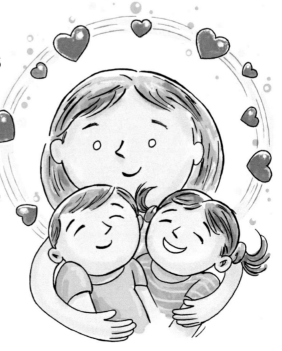

And most of all, remember:

Mummy still loves you and you still love Mummy.

The next three pages have pictures for you to colour in if you would like to! If you are very young, you might want a grown-up to help! The grown-up can also help you name things that you can see in the pictures.

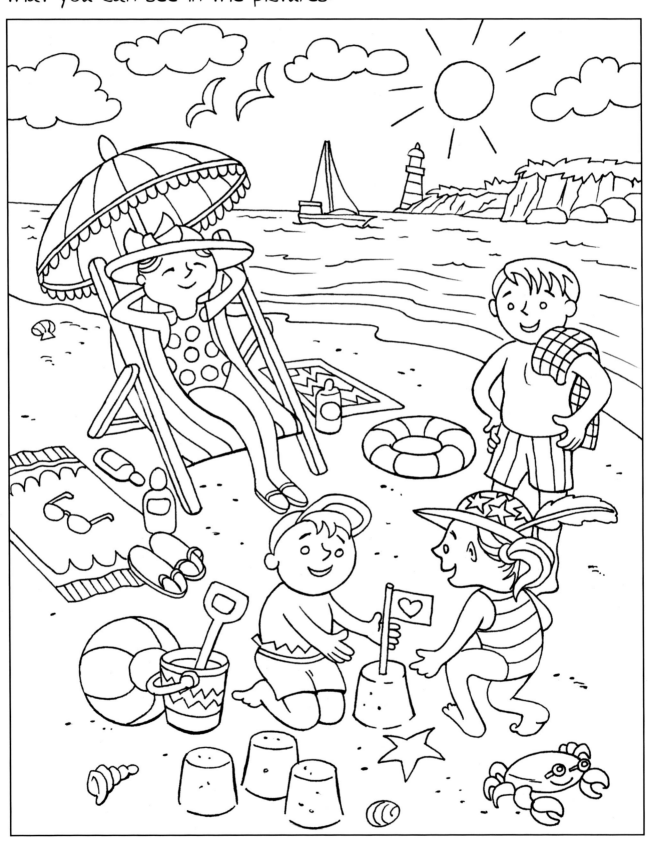

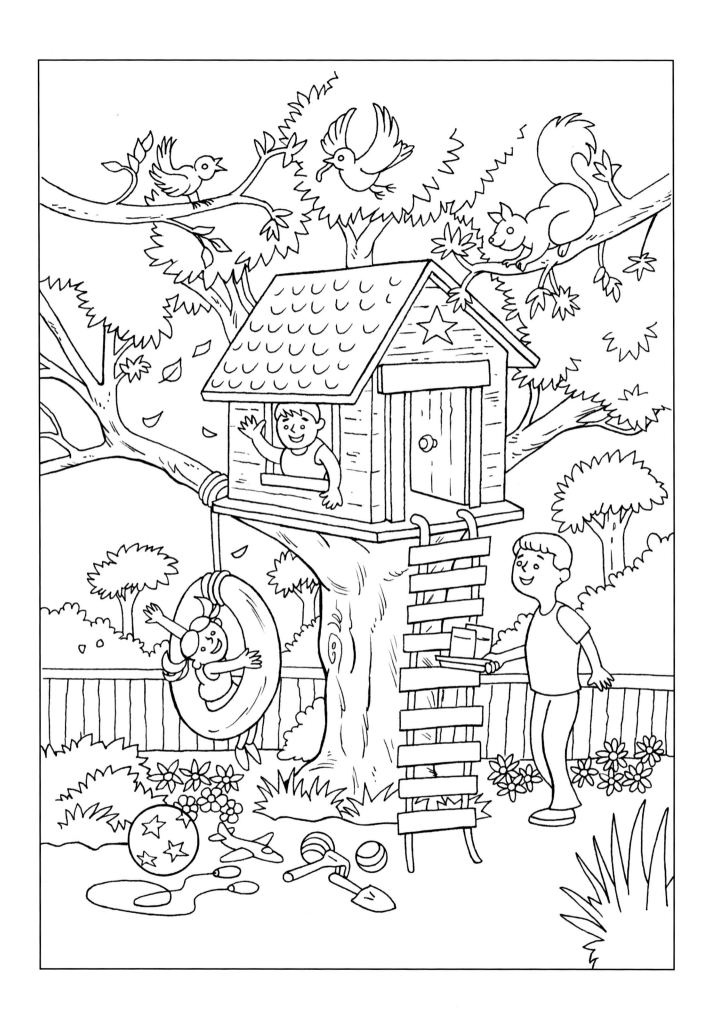

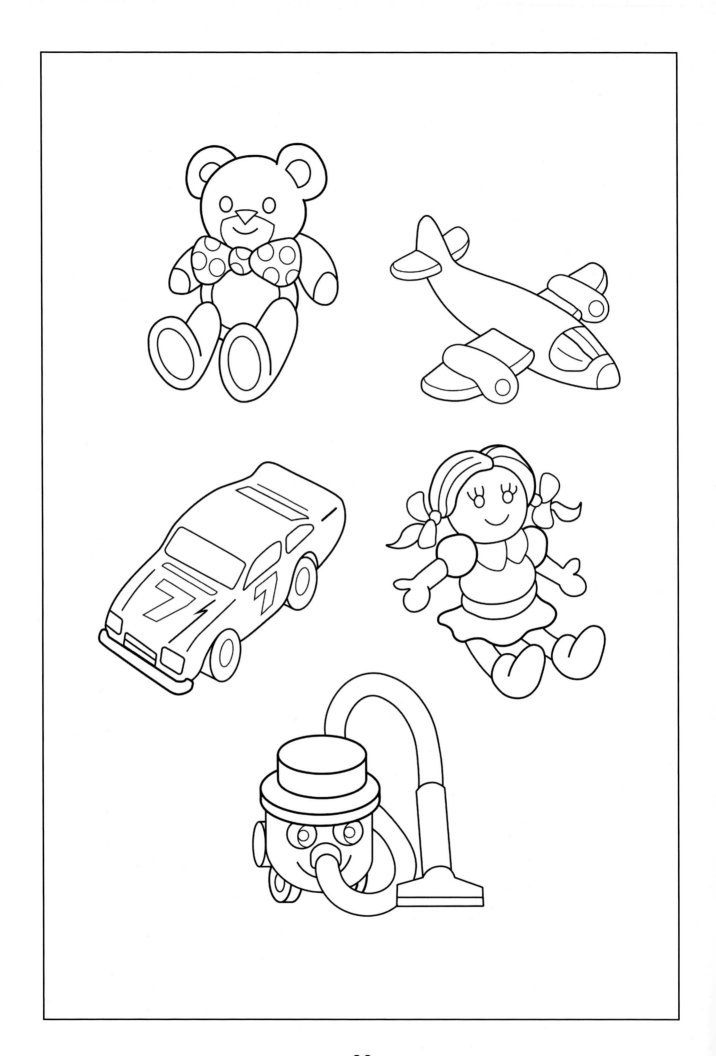

Can you match the feelings on the faces with the words?
Check if you're right by following the strings!

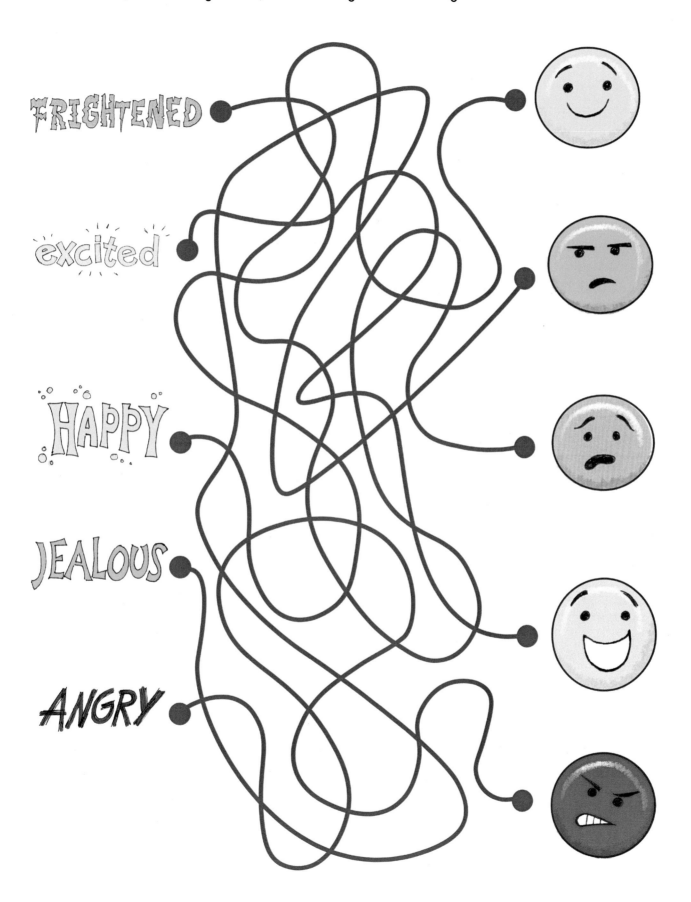

FRIGHTENED

excited

HAPPY

JEALOUS

ANGRY

Can you spot the six differences in the pictures below?

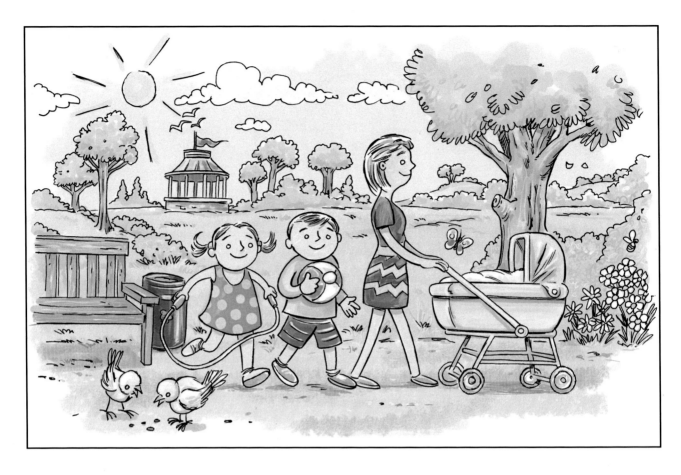

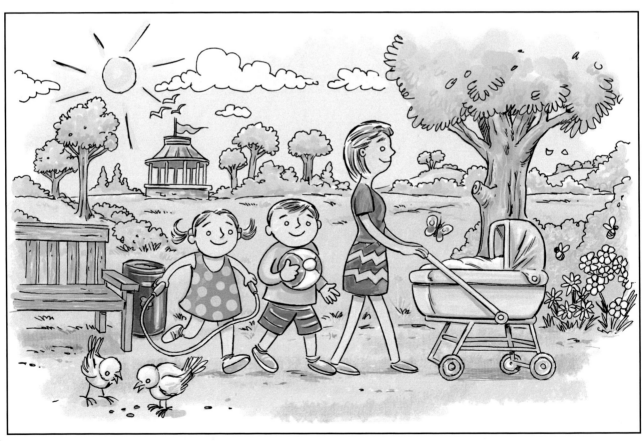

A page for you to stick photos on, or anything else you like!

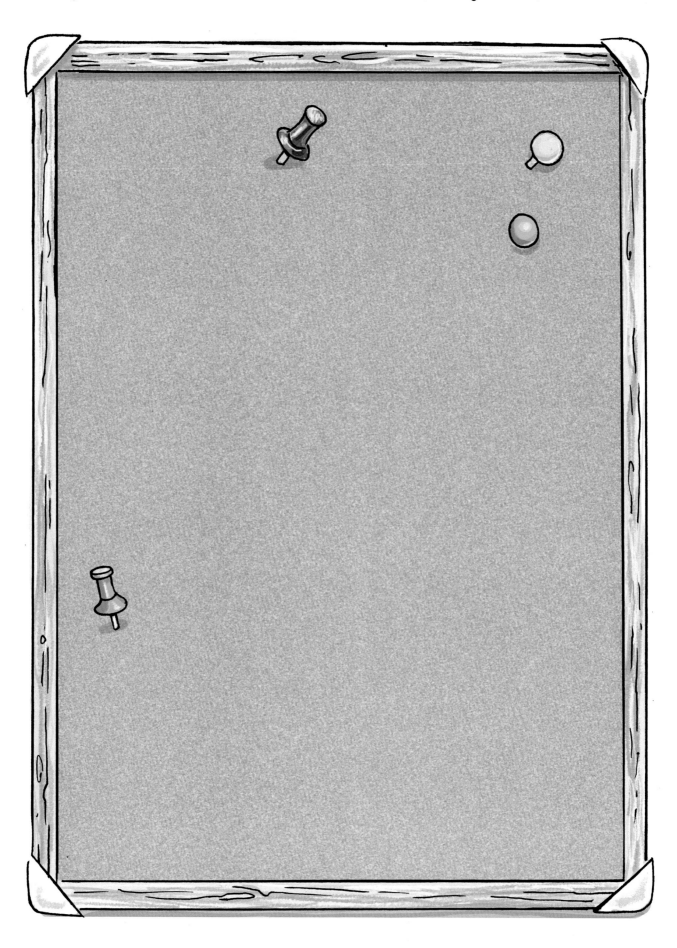

The next four pages are blank for you to draw, colour or write anything you want to.

This book was co-produced by a founding member of www.HampshireLanterns.com and an experienced staff member working within a Perinatal Team after discussions around what parents would have found useful to help support their young children when they had a mental health problem around the time their new baby arrived.

We estimate this book to be useful to children in the age range of 3–9 years. However, all children are different and we have suggested ways of using this book in the introduction to adapt to your child's age and needs.

As part of the profits from this book will be going to charity, we hope that by selling this book we can raise more funds to support parents and their families during difficult times.

We hope you've found it helpful and fun, and would really welcome any feedback (feedback@mymummyand.me).

Printed in the United States
By Bookmasters